RICHA YADAV

The Working Mom's Compass: Finding Your True North in Motherhood and Career

Striking Harmony Between Motherhood and Career: A Guide for the Modern Working Mom

This book was professionally typeset on Reedsy.
Find out more at reedsy.com

"Motherhood has a very humanizing effect. Everything gets reduced to essentials."

Meryl Streep

Contents

1

INTRODUCTION

In the hustle and bustle of modern-day life, the contemporary mom faces a daily struggle that is nothing short of extraordinary. The expectations placed upon her shoulders are numerous and relentless—simultaneously managing a demanding career, maintaining a harmonious home, and nurturing the hearts and minds of her children. It is a perpetual balancing act that, at times, can feel like walking a tightrope suspended over a vast chasm of responsibilities.

The journey of a modern mom is an intricate tapestry woven with threads of ambition, love, sacrifice, and an unyielding commitment to family. The workplace demands proficiency and dedication, requiring her to navigate the complexities of professional growth and fulfillment. Yet, as the clock ticks away during office hours, thoughts of the homefront linger—a mental to-do list filled with groceries to buy, meals to prepare, and the ever-present, delicate needs of her children.

The quest for balance becomes an ardent pursuit, a daily striving to meet the expectations of both the workplace and the home, all while maintaining a semblance of personal well-being.

In this quest, she discovers that the concept of **"having it all"** is a nuanced and elusive ideal, and the pursuit of perfection often comes at the cost of her own mental and physical health.

The overwhelming nature of this juggling act is exacerbated by societal pressures and the pervasive myth of the supermom who effortlessly excels in all areas of life. The modern mom is often left grappling with guilt when she inevitably falls short of these unrealistic standards—guilt for not spending enough quality time with her children, guilt for not achieving professional milestones as swiftly as expected, and guilt for not dedicating more time to self-care.

It is amidst this whirlwind of expectations, responsibilities, and the ceaseless ticking of the clock that the modern mom's struggle comes to the forefront. The pages of her life unfold with moments of chaos and calm, tears and laughter, as she navigates the labyrinth of emotions tied to her roles as a professional, a homemaker, and a mother.

Yet, within this struggle lies resilience, determination, and an unwavering commitment to create a life that encompasses all facets of her identity. In the overwhelm, she embarks on a quest for balance—an earnest endeavor to harmonize the discordant notes of her daily life, finding a rhythm that allows for the fulfillment of her own aspirations, the nurturing of her family, and the preservation of her sanity.

"Balanced Bliss: Navigating Work, Home, and Motherhood" is a testament to the modern mom's journey—a journey marked by struggle, triumph, and the relentless pursuit of equilibrium. It is a narrative that acknowledges the overwhelming nature of her daily existence while providing insights, support, and a sense of solidarity. Through these pages, we explore the intricate dance of a woman who wears many hats, inviting readers to recognize the beauty in the chaos and to find inspiration in the strength of those who dare to juggle the extraordinary demands of the modern-day mom.

2

Chapter 1: Mapping Your Priorities

Identifying Core Values

In the tumultuous journey of modern motherhood, where the demands of work, home, and personal aspirations collide, establishing a firm foundation is paramount. This chapter is an exploration of the bedrock upon which the delicate balancing act is built—the identification of core values that define the essence of your existence.

Navigating the Inner Compass

In the whirlwind of responsibilities, it's easy to lose sight of the principles that guide our decisions and actions. The first step in mapping your priorities is to embark on a journey within, a soul-searching expedition to discern the values that resonate at your core. What matters most to you in the grand tapestry of life? Is it family, career fulfillment, personal growth, or a harmonious blend of these elements?

This section delves into the intricacies of identifying your core values—those fundamental beliefs and principles that shape your identity and govern your choices. Through introspective exercises and thought-provoking reflections, we will unveil the compass that directs your path, illuminating the values that anchor you in times of chaos and guide you towards a life of purpose.

Section 1: Identifying Core Values

In the chaotic landscape of a modern mom's life, identifying core values is akin to finding the North Star in the night sky— a constant guide that provides direction amidst the swirling demands of work, home, and personal aspirations. This section is a deep dive into the methods and reflections that will assist you in unraveling the tapestry of your beliefs and principles.

1.1 Self-Reflection: Looking Inward

Begin the journey by setting aside dedicated time for self-reflection. Find a quiet space where you can contemplate without interruptions. Ask yourself probing questions such as:

- What aspects of my life bring me the most joy and fulfillment?
- When do I feel most aligned with my true self?
- Which moments in my life have left a lasting impact on me?

Through this introspective process, you may discover recurring themes and patterns that point towards your core values. For example, if you find immense joy in spending quality time with your children and family, "Family" might emerge as a core value.

Example 1: The Power of Connection

Sara, a working mom, reflected on her happiest moments and

discovered that the common thread was the sense of connection with others. She realized that "Connection" was a fundamental value for her, influencing her choices in both personal and professional spheres.

1.2 Values Assessment Tools

Consider utilizing values assessment tools or worksheets designed to guide you through a structured process of self-discovery. These tools often present a list of common values, prompting you to select those that resonate most deeply with you. The act of choosing values forces you to prioritize and articulate what truly matters.

Example 2: The Prioritization Process

Anna, a mom juggling a demanding career, used a values assessment tool to prioritize her values. As she reviewed the list, she found herself drawn to "Achievement" and "Balance." This exercise helped her recognize that, despite the challenges, she deeply valued both professional success and a harmonious life.

1.3 Seeking Feedback from Loved Ones

Sometimes, those closest to us can offer valuable insights into our core values. Engage in open conversations with family and friends, seeking their perspectives on what they believe you prioritize in life. Their observations may provide a new lens through which to view your values.

Example 3: Insights from Others

Monika, a mom and wife, discussed her values with her spouse. Surprisingly, her partner highlighted "Adventure" as a key value, noting that Rebecca's love for exploring new places and trying new things was a significant part of who she was.

1.4 Journaling and Mindful Observation

Embark on a journaling journey, documenting your daily experiences, emotions, and reactions. Over time, patterns may emerge, offering clues to the values that consistently surface in various aspects of your life.

Example 4: Discovering Compassion

Sonia, a mom with a demanding career, noticed a recurring theme of compassion in her journal entries. Whether at work or at home, she consistently found herself drawn to situations where she could extend kindness and support to others, revealing "Compassion" as a core value.

Through these methods, you'll uncover the rich tapestry of your core values, providing a solid foundation for the next step in the journey—crafting a personal mission statement that aligns with your authentic self. Remember, this process is dynamic and ongoing, evolving with your experiences and insights. Embrace the journey of self-discovery with openness and curiosity.

The Intersection of Values and Priorities

As a modern mom, the alignment of your values with your priorities becomes a linchpin for balance. How do your core beliefs influence the way you allocate your time and energy? How can you ensure that your actions mirror your deeply held convictions? By understanding the intersection of values and priorities, you lay the groundwork for a life that is not only productive but also deeply fulfilling.

Creating a Personal Mission Statement

With the compass of your core values in hand, the journey continues into the realm of crafting a personal mission statement—a guiding manifesto that encapsulates your purpose, aspirations, and the legacy you wish to leave behind.

Crafting Your Mission: A Declaration of Purpose

In this section, we delve into the art of creating a personal mission statement that serves as a beacon in the chaos. What is the overarching purpose that drives you to navigate the intricate dance of work, home, and motherhood? How can you articulate your aspirations in a concise and powerful statement that becomes your north star?

Through reflective exercises and guided prompts, we explore the elements that contribute to a robust mission statement. From defining your long-term goals to encapsulating your values in succinct language, this process is an opportunity to crystallize your intentions and fortify your resolve in the face of daily challenges.

Aligning Actions with Aspirations

A personal mission statement is not merely a declaration; it is a call to action. In this part of the chapter, we discuss strategies for aligning your daily actions with the aspirations outlined in your mission statement. How can your professional pursuits, family decisions, and personal endeavors harmonize with the essence of your mission? Through intentional planning and mindful decision-making, you can bridge the gap between your ideals and the reality of your daily life.

As we embark on this journey of mapping your priorities, remember that the process is as significant as the destination. Through self-discovery and intentional crafting, you lay the groundwork for a life that is not only balanced but purposeful—a life guided by the compass of your core values and fueled by a mission that reflects the very essence of who you are.

3

Chapter 2: Navigating The Work Landscape

In the intricate dance of work, home, and motherhood, the professional arena becomes a significant stage for the modern working woman. This section is dedicated to the exploration and cultivation of career goals and aspirations—a crucial aspect of the delicate balancing act.

1.1 Defining Your Professional North Star

Begin by envisioning your long-term professional aspirations. What does success look like to you? What impact do you want to make in your career? Define your "professional north star"—a guiding light that illuminates the path toward your career goals.

Example 1: Architecting Ambition

Sophie, a dedicated professional and mother, envisions herself as a leader in her field, spearheading innovative projects that contribute positively to her industry. Her career goal is to be recognized as an influential figure who paves the way for others.

1.2 Balancing Ambition and Realism

While setting ambitious career goals is essential, it's equally important to strike a balance between ambition and realism. Consider the current stage of your life, the demands of your family, and the resources available. Craft goals that are challenging yet achievable within the context of your unique circumstances.

Example 2: Striking the Balance

Emma, a working mom with young children, aspires to climb the corporate ladder. However, she acknowledges the need for a balanced approach that accommodates her family life. Her career goal is to progress steadily while maintaining a work-life harmony that allows her to be present for her children.

1.3 Tailoring Goals to Your Passion

Align your career goals with your passions and areas of expertise. What aspects of your work bring you the most fulfillment? By integrating passion into your professional aspirations, you infuse purpose into your daily endeavors.

Example 3: Fusing Passion with Profession

Laura, a working mom in the field of environmental advocacy, aspires to merge her passion for sustainability with her career. Her goal is to lead projects that drive positive environmental change, creating a meaningful impact aligned with her values.

Section 2: Strategies for Professional Fulfillment

With your career goals and aspirations defined, the next step is to explore strategies for achieving professional fulfillment. This section provides practical insights and approaches to help you navigate the complexities of the professional landscape.

2.1 Embracing Flexibility

In the pursuit of work-life balance, flexibility becomes a key ally. Explore and negotiate flexible work arrangements that allow you to fulfill your professional responsibilities while accommodating the evolving needs of your family.

Example 4: Negotiating Flexibility

Olivia, a working mother of two, negotiated a flexible work schedule that includes remote work options. This flexibility enables her to be present for her children's important moments while excelling in her professional role.

2.2 Building a Supportive Network

Cultivate a professional network that understands and supports your unique challenges as a working mom. Surround yourself with mentors, colleagues, and friends who champion your career goals and provide valuable insights and encouragement.

Example 5: The Power of Networking

Jasmine, a career-oriented mom, actively participates in industry-related events and networking groups. Her supportive network not only offers guidance in navigating professional challenges but also opens doors to new opportunities.

2.3 Continuous Learning and Skill Development

Stay ahead in your field by prioritizing continuous learning and skill development. Invest in professional development opportunities, certifications, and training programs that enhance your expertise and keep you competitive.

Example 6: Lifelong Learning Commitment

Maria, a mother dedicated to her career in technology, consistently engages in online courses and workshops to stay abreast of industry trends. Her commitment to continuous learning positions her as a valuable asset in her professional sphere.

2.4 Goal-oriented Time Management

Efficient time management is a cornerstone of professional fulfillment. Establish clear goals, prioritize tasks, and implement effective time management strategies to maximize productivity both at work and at home.

Example 7: The Power of Prioritization

Rachel, a working mom in a demanding managerial role, prioritizes her daily tasks based on urgency and importance. This goal-oriented time management approach enables her to meet work deadlines while ensuring quality time with her family.

2.5 Seeking Mentorship and Guidance

Explore mentorship opportunities within your industry. A mentor can provide invaluable guidance, share experiences, and offer advice on navigating the complexities of your professional journey.

Example 8: The Mentorship Advantage

Hannah, a working mother aspiring to advance her career, sought mentorship from a senior executive in her company. The guidance received not only accelerated her professional growth but also provided insights into balancing leadership roles with family responsibilities.

2.6 Advocating for Yourself

As a working mom, it's crucial to advocate for yourself in the workplace. Clearly communicate your career goals, express your aspirations, and proactively seek opportunities that align with your professional objectives.

Example 9: Self-Advocacy in Action

Amanda, a mother in a dynamic marketing role, consistently communicates her career goals during performance reviews. By articulating her aspirations, she has successfully secured projects that align with her professional growth trajectory.

Navigating the work landscape as a working mom involves a delicate interplay between ambition, strategy, and a commitment to ongoing growth. By defining clear career goals and implementing effective strategies for professional fulfillment, you pave the way for a successful and fulfilling professional journey while maintaining the delicate balance between work, home, and raising children.

4

Chapter 3: Homefront Chronicles

reating a Comfortable and Functional Living Space In the intricate tapestry of a working mom's life, the home front is the sacred space where the dance of family life unfolds. This section delves into the art of crafting a living environment that nurtures harmony, functionality, and comfort—a haven that supports the delicate balance between work, home, and raising children.

1.1 Designing Your Sanctuary

Begin by envisioning your home as a sanctuary—an oasis of calm amidst the daily hustle. Consider the layout, colors, and elements that bring a sense of tranquility. Tailor your living space to align with your family's needs, creating designated areas for work, play, and relaxation.

Example 1: The Sanctuary Corner

Sophie, a working mom, transformed a corner of her living room into a cozy reading nook. This intentional design element allows her to unwind with a book after work, fostering a sense of calm and rejuvenation.

1.2 Organization as a Pillar

Embrace the power of organization to maintain a functional living space. Implement storage solutions, declutter regularly, and establish routines that streamline daily tasks. An organized home reduces stress, making it easier to navigate the demands of family life.

Example 2: The Power of Decluttering

Emma, a mom with a bustling household, embraced decluttering as a regular practice. By periodically purging unused items and organizing spaces, she created an environment that promotes a sense of order and simplicity.

1.3 Incorporating Personal Touches

Infuse your living space with personal touches that reflect the uniqueness of your family. Whether it's framed photographs, artwork, or sentimental items, these elements contribute to a warm and inviting atmosphere.

Example 3: Personalized Family Gallery

Leena , a working mom, created a family gallery wall in her living room. The wall showcases photographs capturing cherished moments, fostering a sense of connection and warmth within the home.

1.4 Creating Functional Workspaces

If working from home is a part of your routine, carve out functional workspaces that promote productivity. Designate areas for focused work, equipped with the necessary tools and technology, to maintain a clear boundary between professional and personal spaces.

Example 4: The Productivity Nook

Aneeta, a working mom, transformed a corner of her bedroom into a dedicated workspace. By incorporating a desk, ergonomic chair, and good lighting, she created a conducive environment for focused work.

The Mental To-Do List: Juggling Responsibilities for Family and Self

Beyond the tangible aspects of the home, the mental to-do list occupies a significant space in the mind of a working mom. This section explores strategies to navigate the mental juggling act, ensuring that responsibilities for family and self are managed with grace.

2.1 Embracing Mindfulness Practices

Cultivate mindfulness practices to anchor yourself amidst the mental whirlwind. Incorporate moments of meditation, deep breathing, or mindful pauses throughout the day to center your thoughts and reduce mental clutter.

Example 5: Morning Mindfulness Ritual

Manisha, a working mom, starts her day with a brief mindfulness ritual. Before the rush begins, she takes a few minutes to breathe deeply and set positive intentions for the day ahead.

2.2 Prioritizing and Planning

Prioritize tasks and create a structured plan to manage your mental to-do list. Break down larger tasks into manageable steps, set realistic deadlines, and utilize tools like planners or digital apps to stay organized.

Example 6: The Power of Planning

Rachel, a mom in a demanding managerial role, relies on a detailed planner to organize her daily tasks. By prioritizing and planning, she efficiently juggles work commitments, family responsibilities, and personal self-care.

2.3 Delegating and Asking for Help

Recognize the power of delegation and don't hesitate to ask for help when needed. Share responsibilities with family members, create a support network, and communicate openly about your needs to lighten the mental load.

Example 7: Shared Responsibilities

Amanda, a working mom, established a system of shared responsibilities with her spouse. By delegating tasks and openly communicating about their individual capacities, they maintain a balanced division of household duties.

2.4 Setting Realistic Expectations

Manage expectations by setting realistic goals for yourself and your family. Understand that perfection is not the goal; rather, it's about finding a balance that aligns with your values and supports the well-being of your loved ones.

Example 8: Embracing Imperfection

Hannah, a working mom, learned to embrace imperfection and set realistic expectations. By releasing the pressure to achieve perfection in every aspect of life, she created a more relaxed and enjoyable family environment.

2.5 Carving Out Me-Time

Acknowledge the importance of self-care by carving out dedicated "me-time" in your schedule. Whether it's a few minutes of solitude, engaging in a hobby, or practicing self-care rituals, prioritize moments that recharge and rejuvenate your mind.

Example 9: Self-Care Rituals

Mona, a mother dedicated to her career, engages in self-care rituals such as a weekly bath or quiet reading time. These intentional moments of self-care contribute to her mental well-being amidst a busy schedule.

Navigating the homefront chronicles involves a delicate interplay of physical surroundings and mental well-being. By intentionally crafting a comfortable and functional living space and adopting strategies to manage the mental to-do list, working moms can foster an environment that supports their unique journey of balancing work, home, and raising children.

5

Chapter 4: The Juggling Act: Balancing Work and Family Life

In the intricate choreography of a working mom's life, the juggling act of balancing work and family is a nuanced dance. This chapter delves into the two pivotal aspects crucial for a seamless performance: Time Management Strategies and Handling Multiple Roles with Grace.

Section 1: Time Management Strategies

1.1 Prioritizing Tasks and Responsibilities

In the juggling act, time is the most precious ball in the air. Prioritizing tasks is paramount. Identify the most critical responsibilities at work and home, ensuring that your time is allocated to activities that align with your overarching goals.

Example 1: The Priority Pyramid

Seema, a working mom, employs the priority pyramid method. She categorizes tasks into **"must-do," "should-do,"** and **"nice-to-do"** to ensure that essential responsibilities are addressed first, maintaining a balance between professional and family commitments.

1.2 Creating a Structured Schedule

Establishing a structured schedule provides a framework for the juggling act. Define specific time blocks for work, family, and personal activities. A well-organized schedule allows for better control over time and minimizes the risk of dropping any metaphorical balls.

Example 2: The Time-Blocked Calendar

Esha, a working mom with a busy schedule, maintains a time-blocked calendar. Each aspect of her life, from work tasks to family activities, has a designated time slot. This method ensures a disciplined approach to time management.

1.3 The Power of Saying "No"

Learning to say "no" is a formidable skill in the juggling act. Recognize your limits and be selective about the commitments you undertake. Saying "no" when necessary preserves your time and energy for priorities that truly matter.

Example 3: The Art of Saying "No"

Charul, a working mom with a penchant for helping others, realized the importance of saying "no" to additional commitments. By being selective, she ensures that she can fulfill her existing responsibilities effectively.

1.4 Leveraging Technology

In the digital age, technology is a valuable ally. Utilize apps, calendars, and productivity tools to streamline tasks, set reminders, and maintain an organized approach to your schedule.

Example 4: The Digital Command Center

Lavanya, a tech-savvy working mom, uses a digital command center app to manage her tasks and schedule. The app helps her stay on top of deadlines, appointments, and family events, contributing to a more efficient juggling act.

Section 2: Handling Multiple Roles with Grace

2.1 Embracing Flexibility

The juggling act often requires a delicate balance between structure and flexibility. Embrace adaptability, recognizing that unexpected events may alter your plans. A flexible mindset allows you to navigate the twists and turns of the juggling act with grace.

Example 5: The Flexible Planner

Rachel, a working mom managing a dynamic career, cultivates a flexible approach to her plans. While maintaining a structured schedule, she remains adaptable, adjusting her priorities when unforeseen events arise at work or home.

2.2 Establishing Clear Boundaries

Define clear boundaries between work and family roles to prevent the lines from blurring. When engaged in one role, be fully present, avoiding distractions that may hinder your effectiveness in another.

Example 6: The Art of Presence

Smita, a working mom, practices the art of presence. When she's at work, she is fully immersed in her tasks. Similarly, when spending time with her family, she focuses on being present and engaged, fostering a balance between roles.

2.3 Delegating Responsibilities

Recognize that you don't have to juggle all the balls alone. Delegate tasks at work and home, involving family members and colleagues in shared responsibilities. Delegation lightens the load, making the juggling act more sustainable.

Example 7: Shared Responsibilities at Home

Hina, a working mom and spouse, actively involves her family in household responsibilities. By delegating tasks and collaborating with her spouse and children, she creates a supportive environment that eases the juggling act.

2.4 Practicing Self-Compassion

The juggling act can be demanding, and perfection is not the goal. Practice self-compassion, acknowledging that it's okay to drop a ball occasionally. Be forgiving of yourself and recognize the resilience it takes to manage multiple roles.

Example 8: Embracing Imperfection

Mira, a mother dedicated to her career, embraces imperfection. She acknowledges that there will be moments when certain responsibilities take precedence, and that's perfectly fine. Self-compassion is a key element in gracefully handling multiple roles.

Balancing work and family life is an intricate dance, and mastering the juggling act requires a combination of strategic time management and the ability to handle multiple roles with grace. By implementing effective time management strategies and cultivating resilience in handling diverse responsibilities, the working mom can navigate the juggling act with finesse, ensuring harmony in both professional and family spheres.

Section 3: Navigating Societal Pressures and Expectations

In the intricate dance of the juggling act, societal pressures and expectations often loom as silent spectators. This section explores the significance of breaking free from unrealistic

standards and redefining success on your own terms—a pivotal
step in maintaining balance and well-being.

3.1 Breaking Free from Unrealistic Standards

The societal stage can set unrealistic standards for the working mom, dictating what the perfect career, family, and personal life should look like. It's essential to recognize and challenge these unrealistic expectations, understanding that every journey is unique.

Example 9: Embracing Individuality

Ananya, a working mom, found liberation in embracing her individuality. Rather than conforming to external expectations, she defined success based on her values, aspirations, and the unique dynamics of her family.

3.2 The Myth of Supermom

The myth of the supermom—a flawless individual effortlessly managing all aspects of life—can be a heavy burden. It's crucial to dispel this myth and acknowledge that imperfections and challenges are inherent in the juggling act. Embracing vulnerability becomes a strength.

Example 10: Shattering the Supermom Myth

Ojasvi, a working mom, shattered the supermom myth by openly discussing her challenges with a supportive network. By sharing her experiences, she discovered that vulnerability creates connections and fosters a sense of community among working moms.

3.3 Redefining Success in Your Own Terms

Success is a deeply personal concept, and defining it on your own terms is a liberating act. It involves aligning your achievements with your values and acknowledging that success can manifest in various forms, not confined to traditional expectations.

Example 11: A Personal Definition of Success

Isha, a working mom passionate about her career, redefined success as finding fulfillment in both her professional and family roles. She let go of external benchmarks and embraced a definition that resonated with her own aspirations and values.

3.4 Balancing Ambition and Well-Being

Striking a balance between professional ambition and personal well-being is paramount. The juggling act requires a mindful approach to avoid sacrificing mental and physical health in pursuit of external success. Success should be holistic, encompassing both career achievements and personal fulfillment.

Example 12: The Balanced Equation

Kiran, a career-oriented mom, found balance by reevaluating her priorities. She shifted from chasing external recognition to prioritizing well-being. By embracing a balanced equation of ambition and self-care, she achieved a more sustainable and meaningful version of success.

3.5 Celebrating Unconventional Paths

The juggling act often involves navigating unconventional paths that may diverge from societal norms. Celebrate the beauty of forging your own journey, recognizing that there is strength in choosing a path that aligns with your authentic self.

Example 13: The Unconventional Trailblazer

Radhika, a working mom pursuing a non-traditional career, celebrated her unconventional path. By forging her own trail, she discovered a sense of fulfillment that went beyond societal expectations, demonstrating that success can be found in unexpected places.

Navigating societal pressures and expectations is an integral part of the juggling act. By breaking free from unrealistic standards and redefining success on your own terms, the working mom not only liberates herself from unnecessary burdens but also paves the way for a journey that aligns with her authentic aspirations and values. The power lies in embracing individuality, challenging myths, and celebrating the unconventional paths that lead to a fulfilling and harmonious life.

6

Chapter 5: Parenting Principles

In the elaborate mosaic of a working mom's life, the role of a parent weaves a profound narrative. This chapter delves into two essential aspects of parenting principles: Instilling Values in Your Children and Effective Discipline Strategies— keystones in nurturing a foundation of character, resilience, and love within your family.

Section 1: Instilling Values in Your Children
1.1 The Importance of Family Values

Amidst the bustling rhythm of life, family values serve as the guiding melody. Cultivating a set of shared values provides a moral compass for your children, shaping their character and decision-making as they navigate the world.

Example 14: The Pillars of Integrity

Aarav and Aanya, siblings in a bustling household, were raised with a strong emphasis on integrity. Their parents, Raj and Ananya, consistently modeled honesty, compassion, and responsibility, instilling these values as the pillars of their family foundation.

1.2 Modeling Behavior and Character

Children absorb values not just through words but by observing the behavior of their parents. Modeling the character traits and principles you wish to instill fosters a culture of authenticity and integrity within your family.

Example 15: Leading by Example

Rohan, a father and professional, understood the significance of leading by example. His commitment to hard work, kindness, and humility became the blueprint for his children, demonstrating the values he hoped to instill in them.

1.3 Engaging in Open Communication

Instilling values involves fostering open and honest communication. Create a space where your children feel comfortable expressing their thoughts and emotions. Engaging in meaningful conversations allows you to impart values while understanding the perspectives of your children.

Example 16: The Power of Family Talks

Neha, a mother of three, initiated regular family talks where everyone could share their experiences and perspectives. Through these discussions, she imparted values of empathy, respect, and open-mindedness, creating a culture of understanding within her family.

1.4 Encouraging Empathy and Compassion

Teaching children to empathize and show compassion builds a foundation of kindness and social awareness. Encourage them to consider others' feelings, perspectives, and experiences, fostering a sense of empathy that extends beyond familial boundaries.

Example 17: Acts of Kindness

Avni, a working mom, involved her children in acts of kindness, from volunteering at local charities to simple acts of helping neighbors. These experiences nurtured a sense of compassion, instilling the value of giving back to the community.

Section 2: Effective Discipline Strategies

2.1 Understanding the Purpose of Discipline

Discipline is not just about correction; it's about guiding children to make positive choices and learn from their mistakes. Understanding the purpose of discipline helps create an environment where children can grow, learn, and develop a sense of responsibility.

Example 18: Discipline as Guidance

Raj, a father committed to effective discipline, viewed it as a form of guidance. Instead of punitive measures, he engaged his children in discussions about their actions, encouraging them to reflect on the consequences and make informed choices.

2.2 Consistency and Clear Expectations

Consistency and clear expectations provide a structured framework for discipline. Establishing predictable consequences for certain behaviors helps children understand the boundaries, creating a sense of security and stability.

Example 19: The Power of Consistency

Sanya, a mother of twins, maintained consistent expectations for behavior. Whether at home or in public, her children knew the expectations, creating a sense of predictability that contributed to a harmonious family dynamic.

2.3 Positive Reinforcement

Positive reinforcement is a powerful tool in effective discipline. Acknowledging and rewarding positive behavior reinforces the values you aim to instill, motivating children to make choices aligned with those values.

Example 20: Celebrating Achievements

Vikram, a parent emphasizing positive reinforcement, celebrated his children's achievements, big or small. This approach fostered a positive environment where the focus was on growth, effort, and the joy of learning rather than punitive measures.

2.4 Encouraging Responsibility and Accountability

Effective discipline involves teaching children to take responsibility for their actions and be accountable for the consequences. This principle cultivates a sense of ownership and empowers children to make thoughtful decisions.

Example 21: Learning Accountability

Meera, a working mom, encouraged her children to participate in decision-making processes. By involving them in choices related to their activities and responsibilities, she fostered accountability and a sense of ownership in their actions.

2.5 Time-Outs and Reflection

Time-outs serve as a valuable strategy for children to reflect on their behavior. Instead of being punitive, time-outs offer a moment of introspection, allowing children to understand the impact of their actions on themselves and others.

Example 22: The Reflection Corner

Arjun, a parent who embraced time-outs, designated a reflection corner in the house. When his children needed a moment to collect themselves, they would retreat to this space to reflect and then engage in a constructive discussion.

Navigating the delicate terrain of parenting principles involves a harmonious blend of instilling values and employing effective discipline strategies. By cultivating a culture of shared values within your family and embracing discipline as a form of guidance, you lay the groundwork for character development, resilience, and a loving familial bond.

7

Chapter 6: Communication in the Chaos

In the tumultuous currents of a full and demanding life, the ability to navigate and maintain meaningful connections with our closest loved ones becomes paramount. This chapter delves into the intricacies of Communication in the Chaos, focusing on two pivotal aspects: Nurturing Relationships with Spouse and Children, and Managing Expectations through Effective Communication.

Section 1: Nurturing Relationships with Spouse and Children

1.1 Prioritizing Quality Time

In the whirlwind of daily responsibilities, carving out quality time for your spouse and children is an investment in the heart of your family. Prioritize moments of connection, whether it's a quiet dinner together, a weekend outing, or simply sharing stories before bedtime. Quality time reinforces the bonds that sustain you through life's chaos.

1.2 Cultivating Open and Honest Dialogue

Effective communication within a family is built on a foundation of openness and honesty. Encourage a culture where everyone feels free to express their thoughts and emotions. Cultivating a safe space for dialogue fosters understanding and strengthens the fabric of familial relationships.

1.3 Active Listening in Family Dynamics

Within the chaos of family life, practicing active listening becomes a linchpin for harmonious relationships. Listen not only to the words spoken but also to the nuances of feelings and concerns. Actively engaging in the communication process demonstrates respect and deepens connections.

1.4 Celebrating Milestones Together

Amidst the chaos, take moments to collectively celebrate milestones, whether big or small. Acknowledging achievements, birthdays, and special occasions strengthens the family bond. Shared celebrations create lasting memories and serve as anchors in the midst of life's constant flux.

Section 2: Managing Expectations through Effective Communication

2.1 Setting Clear Expectations

Communication plays a pivotal role in managing expectations within a family. Clearly articulate expectations regarding responsibilities, commitments, and personal boundaries. Setting transparent expectations reduces misunderstandings and promotes a collaborative approach to shared responsibilities.

2.2 Collaborative Decision-Making

In the chaos of family life, decisions are often abundant and varied. Embrace a collaborative approach to decision-making. Engage family members in discussions, gather perspectives, and make choices collectively. This not only strengthens familial bonds but also ensures that everyone feels heard and valued.

2.3 Communicating Changes and Adjustments

Life is dynamic, and changes are inevitable. Effective communication is crucial when navigating transitions, be it a shift in schedules, a change in responsibilities, or adjustments to family routines. Transparently communicating changes helps everyone adapt with understanding and cooperation.

2.4 Expressing Needs and Seeking Support

Encourage family members to express their needs and seek support when necessary. In the chaos of daily life, being attuned to each other's challenges and offering assistance fosters a sense of teamwork. Effective communication becomes a lifeline in creating a supportive family environment.

2.5 Practicing Flexibility and Adaptability

Communicate the importance of flexibility and adaptability within the family unit. Life's chaos often brings unexpected challenges, and the ability to adapt requires open communication and a willingness to adjust expectations. Embracing change together strengthens family resilience.

Navigating the chaos of life involves consciously fostering meaningful connections with your spouse and children. By prioritizing quality time, cultivating open dialogue, and actively engaging in family dynamics, you contribute to a supportive and harmonious familial environment. Simultaneously, effective communication becomes a powerful tool in managing expectations—setting clear boundaries, making decisions collaboratively, and adapting to life's inevitable changes. Through these practices, you create a resilient and connected family unit that thrives amidst the chaos of modern life.

8

Chapter 7: Self-Care for the Super-Mom

In the whirlwind of responsibilities that define the modern mom's life, self-care is not a luxury but a necessity. This chapter delves into the importance of personal well-being and offers practical and easily achievable methods for incorporating self-care into your daily routine.

1. Importance of Personal Well-Being

1.1 Recognizing the Superpower of Self-Care

In the demanding role of a super-mom, personal well-being is your superpower. Acknowledge that taking care of yourself is not selfish but a vital component of sustaining the energy and resilience needed for the myriad tasks you juggle daily.

1.2 The Ripple Effect on Family Dynamics

Understand the profound impact your well-being has on your family. A well-nurtured mom is better equipped to handle challenges, provide emotional support, and foster a positive atmosphere at home. Prioritizing self-care is an investment in the overall well-being of your family.

1.3 Balancing the Care Equation

Just as you care for your family, extend that same level of care to yourself. Balancing the care equation involves recognizing your needs, setting boundaries, and allocating time for activities that replenish your physical, mental, and emotional reserves.

2. Incorporating Self-Care into Daily Life

2.1 Mindful Moments in Hectic Schedules

In the hustle of daily life, find moments of mindfulness. Whether it's a few minutes of deep breathing, a mindful walk, or a moment of reflection, these pauses rejuvenate your mind and enhance your ability to navigate the challenges of the day.

2.2 Embracing the Power of "No"

Recognize the strength in saying "no" when necessary. Setting boundaries and managing commitments prevent burnout. Embracing the power of "no" allows you to prioritize activities that align with your well-being and values.

2.3 The Joy of Movement

Incorporate physical activity into your routine, even in small doses. Whether it's a brief workout, a dance session in the living room, or a brisk walk, movement releases endorphins and contributes to both physical and mental well-being.

2.4 Creating Personal Retreats at Home

Designate spaces at home as personal retreats. These can be cozy corners for reading, meditation nooks, or simply spaces where you can unwind. Having designated areas for relaxation contributes to a sense of sanctuary within your own home.

2.5 Nourishing Nutrition for Energy

Prioritize nourishing your body with wholesome foods. Even in the midst of a busy schedule, make conscious choices to fuel your body with the nutrients it needs. Balanced nutrition contributes not only to physical well-being but also to sustained energy levels.

2.6 Prioritizing Sleep as a Non-Negotiable

Recognize the non-negotiable importance of sleep. Quality rest is foundational to overall well-being. Establish healthy sleep habits, create a calming bedtime routine, and ensure you allocate sufficient time for a restful night's sleep.

2.7 Cultivating Hobbies for Joyful Expression

Incorporate hobbies that bring joy and creative expression into your life. Whether it's reading, painting, gardening, or any other passion, engaging in activities you love contributes to a sense of fulfillment and joy.

2.8 Connecting with Supportive Networks

Foster connections with supportive networks. Share experiences, seek advice, and lean on friends and family when needed. Building a network of understanding individuals creates a supportive community that enhances your well-being.

3. Embracing Self-Care as an Essential Practice

3.1 Dispelling Guilt and Prioritizing Yourself

Release any guilt associated with prioritizing your well-being. Understand that self-care is not a selfish act but a necessary practice for your own health and the well-being of your family. Prioritizing yourself is an act of strength and self-love.

3.2 Crafting a Personalized Self-Care Routine

Tailor your self-care routine to align with your preferences and lifestyle. Whether it's a daily ritual, a weekly indulgence, or spontaneous moments of self-pampering, create a routine that resonates with you and is easily integrated into your daily life.

3.3 Celebrating Progress, Not Perfection

Acknowledge that self-care is a continuous journey, not a destination. Celebrate the progress you make in incorporating self-care into your life, recognizing that small, consistent steps lead to lasting well-being.

In the modern era, the super-mom of today must recognize the importance of personal well-being and integrate self-care practices seamlessly into her daily routine. By embracing self-care as a non-negotiable aspect of a fulfilling life, you not only nurture your own well-being but also contribute to a healthier, happier, and more harmonious family environment.

4.1 Navigating Mom's Guilt: Finding Grace in Imperfection

4.1.1 Understanding the Roots of Mom's Guilt

Mom's guilt often stems from the perceived gap between expectations and reality. Understand that these expectations are often influenced by societal standards and self-imposed ideals. Recognizing the source of guilt is the first step towards navigating it.

4.1.2 Cultivating Self-Compassion

Replace self-judgment with self-compassion. Acknowledge that being a super-mom doesn't mean being perfect. Embrace the reality of imperfection, and let self-compassion be the antidote to mom's guilt. Treat yourself with the same kindness and understanding you extend to others.

4.1.3 Celebrating Small Wins

Shift the focus from perceived shortcomings to small victories. Celebrate the daily accomplishments, no matter how minor. By acknowledging your efforts and successes, you redirect your attention away from guilt towards positive reinforcement.

4.2 Guilt & Grace: Finding Solace in Imperfection

4.2.1 Embracing the Beauty of Imperfection

Understand that imperfection is not a flaw but a beautiful aspect of being human. Embrace the messiness of life and parenthood, recognizing that the journey is filled with highs and lows. Finding solace in imperfection allows you to release guilt and welcome grace.

4.2.2 Redefining Success in Parenthood

Challenge conventional definitions of successful parenting. Success doesn't equate to flawlessness; it's about love, connection, and the effort you invest. By reframing your understanding of success, you free yourself from the shackles of mom's guilt and open the door to grace.

4.2.3 Setting Realistic Expectations

Adjust expectations to align with reality. Recognize that being a super-mom doesn't mean having it all together all the time.

Set realistic expectations for yourself and your family, fostering an environment where imperfections are acknowledged and embraced.

4.3 Coping with the Emotional Labyrinth

4.3.1 Validating Emotions without Judgment

Embrace the spectrum of emotions that come with motherhood. Validate your feelings without judgment, recognizing that a range of emotions is a natural part of the journey. Allow yourself the space to feel and express, acknowledging that emotional complexity is inherent in parenting.

4.3.2 Establishing Emotional Boundaries

Establish clear emotional boundaries to protect your well-being. Understand that you can support and empathize with your children without absorbing their emotions entirely. Creating emotional boundaries fosters resilience and prevents being overwhelmed by the emotional labyrinth of parenthood.

4.3.3 Seeking Support and Connection

Connect with other moms and build a support network. Share your experiences, challenges, and emotions with trusted friends or support groups. Knowing that you're not alone in navigating the emotional labyrinth provides validation and strengthens your emotional resilience.

4.3.4 Prioritizing Emotional Self-Care

Incorporate emotional self-care into your routine. Whether it's journaling, meditation, or engaging in activities that bring joy, prioritize moments that nurture your emotional well-being. Emotional self-care equips you with the tools to navigate the intricate maze of emotions.

4.4 The Path to Graceful Motherhood

4.4.1 Embracing the Journey, Not Just the Destination

Shift the focus from reaching an idealized destination to embracing the ongoing journey of motherhood. Recognize that growth, learning, and transformation occur throughout the entire process. Embracing the journey allows you to navigate challenges with resilience and grace.

4.4.2 Balancing Responsibilities with Self-Care

Acknowledge the delicate balance between responsibilities and self-care. Understand that prioritizing your well-being isn't selfish but a necessary component of being a present and nurturing mother. Balancing responsibilities with self-care contributes to a harmonious and graceful motherhood.

4.4.3 Choosing Grace Over Perfection

In every moment, choose grace over perfection. Understand that grace allows for flexibility, self-compassion, and the acceptance of imperfections. By choosing grace, you navigate the complexities of motherhood with resilience, love, and an open heart.

In the realm of self-care for the super-mom, navigating mom's guilt, embracing imperfection, and coping with the emotional labyrinth are integral aspects of nurturing your well-being. By understanding the roots of guilt, finding solace in imperfection, and establishing emotional boundaries, you pave the way for a journey marked by grace, resilience, and the beauty of imperfect motherhood.

9

Chapter 8: Strategies for a Harmonious Home

In the bustling hub of family life, cultivating a harmonious home is the cornerstone of a thriving family dynamic. This chapter explores practical strategies for achieving harmony amidst the chaos, focusing on three key pillars: Delegating Responsibilities, Creating a Supportive Network, and Celebrating Triumphs Amidst the Turmoil.

1. Importance of Delegating Responsibilities

1.1 Sharing the Load

Understand that managing a household is a team effort. Delegate tasks and responsibilities among family members, fostering a sense of shared ownership and collaboration. By distributing tasks equitably, you alleviate the burden on yourself and cultivate a spirit of teamwork.

1.2 Teaching Independence

Empower your children by involving them in household responsibilities. Assign age-appropriate tasks and encourage them to take initiative. Teaching independence not only lightens your load but also instills valuable life skills in your children, fostering their sense of competence and self-reliance.

2. Creating a Supportive Network

2.1 Cultivating Relationships

Nurture relationships with friends, family, and neighbors who provide support and encouragement. Cultivating a supportive network creates a safety net during challenging times and offers opportunities for shared experiences and resources.

2.2 Seeking Help When Needed

Recognize that it's okay to ask for help. Reach out to your support network when feeling overwhelmed or in need of assistance. Whether it's childcare, emotional support, or practical help, lean on your network to navigate the ups and downs of parenthood with greater ease.

3. Celebrating Triumphs Amidst the Turmoil

3.1 Embracing Small Victories

Amidst the chaos of daily life, celebrate small triumphs and milestones. Recognize and acknowledge the accomplishments, no matter how minor. Embracing small victories fosters a positive atmosphere and reinforces the resilience and perseverance within your family.

3.2 Cultivating Gratitude

Practice gratitude as a family. Encourage expressions of appreciation and acknowledgment for the blessings and joys in your lives. Cultivating gratitude shifts the focus from challenges to blessings, fostering a sense of contentment and well-being amidst the turmoil.

3.3 Rituals of Celebration

Incorporate rituals of celebration into your family routine. Whether it's a weekly family dinner, a monthly game night, or an annual tradition, create opportunities to come together and celebrate as a family. These rituals strengthen bonds and create lasting memories amidst life's tumultuous moments.

4. The Path to a Harmonious Home

In the pursuit of a harmonious home, remember that it's the collective effort and shared experiences that shape the family dynamic. By delegating responsibilities, creating a supportive network, and celebrating triumphs amidst the turmoil, you pave the way for a home filled with love, resilience, and joy. Together, as a family, you navigate parenthood with ease and grace, fostering a harmonious environment where each member thrives and flourishes.

10

Chapter 9: Thriving in Transition

Life is a journey marked by transitions, each presenting its own set of challenges and opportunities. This chapter explores strategies for thriving amidst change, focusing on two vital aspects: Managing Life Changes and Embracing Flexibility in Your Plans.

1. Managing Life Changes: New Jobs, Moves, and Family Additions

1.1 Embracing the Unknown

Transitions often bring uncertainty, but they also offer opportunities for growth and new beginnings. Embrace the unknown with an open mind and a spirit of curiosity. Approach life changes as adventures waiting to unfold, rather than challenges to be feared.

1.2 Planning and Preparation

While embracing the unknown, it's also important to plan and prepare for transitions. Anticipate potential challenges and create strategies to address them proactively. Whether it's researching a new location, setting up support systems, or creating a financial plan, preparation eases the transition process.

1.3 Seeking Support and Guidance

During times of change, don't hesitate to seek support and guidance from trusted friends, family, or professionals. Surround yourself with a supportive network that can offer encouragement, practical advice, and emotional support as you navigate life's transitions.

2. Embracing Flexibility in Your Plans

2.1 Letting Go of Rigidity

Flexibility is key to navigating life's twists and turns. Let go of rigid expectations and embrace the fluidity of life. Understand that plans may need to be adjusted along the way, and be open to exploring alternative paths that may lead to unexpected opportunities.

2.2 Adapting to New Circumstances

When life throws unexpected curveballs, be prepared to adapt and pivot. Instead of resisting change, view it as an opportunity for growth and learning. Adaptability allows you to navigate challenges with resilience and creativity, turning obstacles into stepping stones for progress.

2.3 Practicing Mindfulness and Presence

In the midst of transitions, practice mindfulness and presence. Stay grounded in the present moment, allowing yourself to fully experience and process the changes unfolding around you. Mindfulness cultivates a sense of calm and clarity, enabling you to make decisions from a place of centeredness.

3. The Path to Thriving in Transition

In the journey of life, transitions are inevitable. By embracing change with grace and flexibility, you not only navigate transitions more smoothly but also thrive amidst the uncertainty. Through careful planning, seeking support, and embracing adaptability, you harness the power of transitions to grow, evolve, and create a life filled with resilience, purpose, and joy

11

Chapter 10: Nurturing Your Career and Family Future

In the journey of life, balancing career aspirations with family responsibilities is like tending to a garden—requiring careful nurturing and planning. This chapter focuses on two essential aspects: Financial Planning for the Modern Family and Balancing Long-Term Goals with Daily Realities, offering practical insights in easy-to-understand style.

1. Financial Planning for the Modern Family

1.1 Making Money Make Sense

Begin by getting a clear picture of your family's financial goals. Think about big things like buying a home, saving for your kids' education, and planning for retirement. Having a roadmap helps you steer in the right direction.

1.2 Keeping Track of Coins and Cents

Create a budget that matches your goals and what's important to your family. Look at where your money goes each month, find ways to save a bit here and there, and put money aside for saving and investing. It's like putting pennies in a piggy bank for a rainy day.

1.3 Putting Your Money to Work

Explore different ways to invest your hard-earned cash. Think about stocks, bonds, property, or special savings accounts for retirement. By spreading your investments out, you're like a smart gardener planting a variety of seeds for a bountiful harvest.

2. Balancing Long-Term Goals with Daily Realities

2.1 Making a To-Do List for Tomorrow and Beyond

Think about your long-term dreams while keeping your feet firmly on the ground. Break down those big goals into smaller steps you can take each day. It's like building a ladder—one step at a time gets you closer to the top.

*2.2 Being Flexible with Your Plans**

Life can throw curveballs, so it's important to have a plan that can bend and flex when needed. Unexpected things can pop up, good and bad, so having a plan that can adjust is like having an umbrella for a rainy day or sunscreen for a sunny one.

2.3 Finding Time for What Matters Most

Learn to manage your time wisely. Set aside moments each day to work towards your goals. It's like watering your plants a little bit every day instead of all at once. Consistency helps things grow steadily.

3. The Path to a Brighter Tomorrow

In nurturing both your career and family future, financial planning and balancing goals with daily life are like the sun and rain for your garden—they help things grow strong and healthy. By setting financial goals, budgeting smartly, and making flexible plans, you're like a gardener with a green thumb, ensuring a fruitful and flourishing future for you and your loved ones. With patience, perseverance, and a little bit of planning, you can cultivate a tomorrow filled with abundance, security, and happiness.

12

Conclusion: Embracing Your Journey and Empowering Fellow Moms

As we come to the end of this insightful journey through the intricacies of balancing work, life, and motherhood, let us take a moment to reflect on two important themes: Celebrating Your Unique Journey and Empowering Fellow Moms to Find Balance.

Celebrate Your Unique Journey

Dear reader, your journey is a tapestry woven with the threads of determination, resilience, and love. Each twist and turn, each triumph and setback, has shaped you into the remarkable woman you are today. Take pride in your journey, in the hurdles you've overcome, and the milestones you've achieved. Celebrate the small victories and the moments of joy, for they are the colors that paint the canvas of your life.

Empower Fellow Moms to Find Balance

As you navigate the complexities of modern motherhood, extend a hand to lift and empower other moms walking a similar path. Share your experiences, your insights, and your support with those who may be struggling to find their balance amidst the chaos. Together, we can create a community of strength, resilience, and solidarity, where every mom feels supported, understood, and empowered to thrive.

In Conclusion

Dear modern-era mom, as you close the chapter on this book, remember that you are not alone in your journey. You are part of a sisterhood of mothers who understand the challenges and joys of balancing work, life, and family. May you find solace in the knowledge that you are doing your best, and that your efforts are seen and appreciated. And may you continue to walk this path with grace, compassion, and the unwavering belief in your ability to conquer whatever challenges come your way. You are strong, you are capable, and you are enough. Here's to you, and to all the incredible moms out there, navigating the beautiful chaos of motherhood with courage and grace.

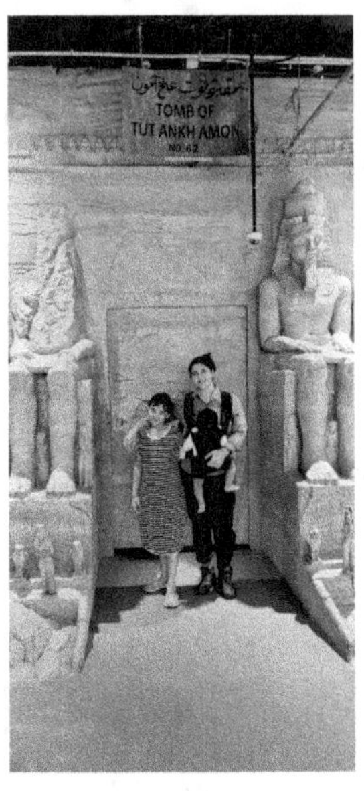

About the Author

Richa Yadav is a soldier, a mother, and a devoted wife who faces life's challenges with unyielding resilience. As an army officer often separated from her husband due to military postings, she grapples with the complexities of balancing her roles. Despite enduring periods of separation and adversity, she remains steadfast in her commitment to her family and her career. In her debut book, **"The Working Mom's Compass: Finding Your True North in Motherhood and Career,"** she candidly shares her personal struggles and empowering strategies for fellow supermoms navigating similar obstacles. With authenticity and perseverance, she invites readers to find strength and inspiration in her journey of resilience and growth.